#TheJumpRopeDiet

http://workoutkingrule.blogspot.com/

workoutkingrule@gmail.com

Checkout

The Sprint Diet: 3 Min Weight Loss HIIT Training

The Kettlebell Cleanse Lose 3600 Calories Ah Day

My Story

My story isn't anything special. My doctor told me I would be a pre-diabetic if I didn't lose weight. Naturally I was a little ashamed because I was a young man at the time. Surprisingly no one told me I had a weight problem. For some reason I was oblivious to it. Looking back on my pictures now I think to myself how didn't I see it. Sometimes we get so comfortable with our bad habits that we don't even see the negative effects. It's similar to how an alcoholic can't see how he's harming himself, and everyone around him. It's similar to how a drug addict can't see that his addiction is deteriorating his appearance.

The day my doctor told me I was in danger of becoming a diabetic changed my life. On that day I decided that my health was more important than my cravings. I decided that my health was more important than my comfortable laziness. Comfort is a funny thing because comfort creates habits. I was comfortable with my negative habits because of that I sacrificed my health. Finding out I was going to be a diabetic was very painful for me. I remember as a child watching my grandmother die of diabetes. I promised her I would take care of myself. I felt like I let her down. I had to do something about my health. I had to do something about my mindset.

In the course of watching some positive, and uplifting videos I came across Muhammad Ali training. I saw his intensity with the jump rope, and I admired it. I could see his speed, and coordination came from his jump roping. Jump roping gave him his ability to dodge so easily. It was the reason he could float like a butterfly, and sting like ah bee. I decided to give it a try. Really what did I have to lose? I immediately figured out that I was no good at it. I loved the workout, but I hated the Rope. I felt like the rope was unnecessary. The majority of the workout is calves, and ankles. So I decided to do a little research to see if it would matter or not if I remove the rope from the equation. Turns out it's not a very big deal as long as you have something in your hand that's just as heavy as the rope handle. I used hand grippers. You've probably seen them before. Just in case you haven't here's a picture.

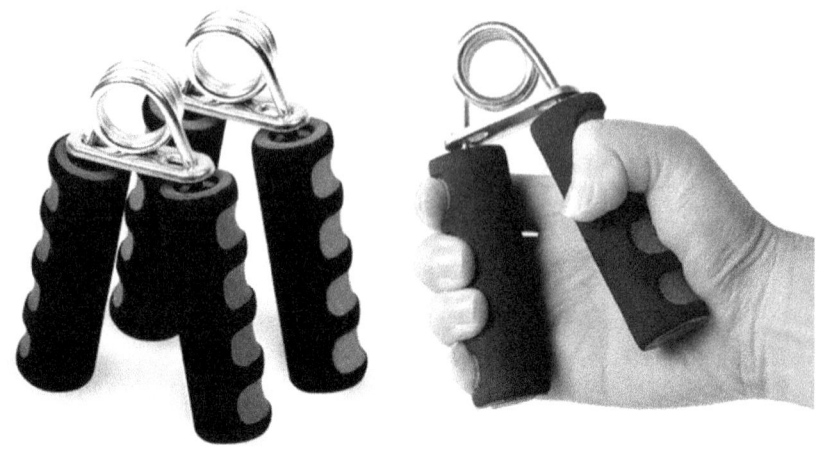

I grab one of the handles on each hand gripper an act like I'm spinning a rope. I even time my jump as if a rope is actually coming down. This exercise helped me burn so much fat in such a short period of time. It's such an easy exercise to do. It's very difficult for me to make excuses not to do it. Plus I couldn't argue with the results. Without the jump rope diet I would have never lost the weight. To believe that something I used to do in Elementary would benefit me later on in life. It was quite surprising to me that I never thought to do it before. I mean if I jumped from the beginning I would've never gained weight in the first place.

I jumped rope for about three to four months. I went to see my doctor, and I got a clean bill of health. I felt like I accomplished something. Even getting my high school diploma, and college degree didn't affect me like that did. This accomplishment felt spiritual mental, and physical. It was such a crazy combination of emotions to hear that news. My wife was proud of me, and I was proud of her. We did this together. When we started we were just dating, and after it was done we were married. I think the journey connected us, and that's why I recommend that you do this with someone else. It doesn't have to be a girlfriend or boyfriend, but the camaraderie really increases everyone's focus.

That was some time ago jump roping has been a part of my life for years now. It's something I do everyday. I should say it's something my wife, and I do everyday. _The Jump Rope Diet_ has been amazing for us, and I know it's going to be amazing for you.

The Benefits Of Jumping Rope

Jump roping Burns anywhere from 10 to 16 calories per minute. Yes I said 10 to 16 calories per minute! That's absolutely astounding! If you keep a steady pace, and really push yourself you can burn a thousand calories every hour using the jump rope. With *The Jump Rope Diet* you don't have to use an actual jump rope. It's a lot easier to continue to work out when you don't have to worry about the rope smacking up against your legs. You're more worried about actually jumping so you can focus.

10 minutes of jump roping is equivalent to ah 8-minute mile. That's absolutely crazy when you think about it. We're talking about a playground exercised out doing the mile run one of the most famous forms of training there is. The mile run is going to put extreme stress on your joints, and it's going to be insanely tiring. Jump roping for 10 minutes isn't going to be nearly as brutal, but just as effective. The American Heart Association has placed its whole movement around jumping rope. Everyone's heard of *Jump Rope for Heart*. When it comes to the fight against heart disease no exercise is more effective than

jumping rope. Jump roping gets your heart rate up everyone knows this. Jump roping promotes a healthy blood flow, and lowers your cholesterol. Jump roping prevents heart disease, and stroke two illnesses that take out some of our best, and brightest. Jump roping strengthens the connection between your body, and your brain. You're jumping on the balls of your feet so your mind has to make neuromuscular adjustments. It does this to make sure that you remain balanced. As this connection gets stronger your body reacts quicker to different situations. It increases the speed in which signals between the body, and the mind can be sent causing you to have quicker reflexes. This is why boxers jump rope because they want to increase their reflexes. Boxes need to be able to move out of the way at any given point in time to avoid injury. By jump roping they develop a strong connection between body and mind. This is why the best boxers in the world are some of the most hardcore jump ropers. Muhammad Ali, and Floyd Mayweather are two of the greatest defensive fighters ever, and they're amazing jump ropers.

Jump roping is great for increasing bone density. Most people think jump roping has a hard impact on your joints, and bones. Jump roping is far less impactful than running. That's because you're landing on both feet. When you run you land on one foot. This puts all the force on one leg. When you jump rope both legs are absorbing the force. Also you're not coming nearly as high off the ground. I only jump an inch to in half an inch off the ground. It's really about the surface that you're jumping on more than anything. I don't jump on concrete. I don't jump on grass. I don't jump on wood! I only jump on carpet with my folded yoga mat under me. I make the surface as soft as I possibly can. I've never had a problem with my knees, ankles, or hips.

Before you start *The Jump Rope Diet* make sure you do some reverse calf raises. Build strength in the muscles most impacted by jump roping. Most likely those muscles are going to be very weak which is where the initial soreness is going to come from. That's why it's good to isolate, and work those muscles with calf raises, and reverse calf raises.

The Jump Rope Diet zaps weight off your body while increasing your focus, and coordination. When you take the rope out of the situation it's an extremely easy exercise. It's something you can do anywhere with virtually zero equipment. Without the rope you don't have to worry about hitting things or knocking things over. You only need body space. You can do it anywhere that has enough space for you to jump an inch to a half an inch off the ground. This made it very easy for me, and my wife. We were able to travel, and go wherever we wanted to without worrying about having enough space to exercise. We literally could exercise in the shower if we wanted to. Not that we did, but we could have. The shower has plenty space for *The Jump Rope Diet*.

Beginners

I'm going to tell you everything that I did in detail. I'll try to make sure I don't leave anything out. Even the smallest details are going to be mentioned so just bear with me. Every morning my wife would get up, and put on motivational workout videos. For some reason those videos motivate her. I'm not talking about videos where people are taking you through a designated workout. It was just a mixture of female fitness models training. At first I didn't really get it, but eventually it did end up motivating me. Something about watching those girls really commit to extreme fitness like CrossFit was motivational. So I didn't bother my wife about it. Now days even when she's not with me I still watch the videos.

Next I fill up a gallon of water. That's right I said a gallon of water! This kind of exercise is going to require you to stay extremely hydrated.

Next I grab my yoga mat, and lay down on the carpet folding it in half.

Next I grabbed my hand grippers.

Now I do this with my socks on I don't wear shoes, but you can if you want. When I was on a beginner level I set my timer to 15 minutes I pressed go, and started jumping as fast as I could. I made sure I only came an inch to ah half an inch off the mat. I have perfect posture making sure not to lean forward or backward. I kept my hands at my side, and I move the hand grippers like I was holding a jump rope. Sometimes I would grab both handles on the hand grippers, and start squeezing them to get a quick wrist, and forearm workout while keeping the turning motion. I would squeeze it about 50 times.

When the timer hit 30 seconds I would stop. Eventually I was able to work myself up to one minute which is what I consider beginner level. When you begin training do 30 sets of 30-second jumps that's 15 minutes. When you gain more stamina you'll go up to 30 sets of one-minute jumps for 30 minutes of exercise. That's what I consider beginner level training. If you can jump longer than by all means do so. Most people will start off on this level. They won't be able to do one-minute jumps right away. If you're the exception than be proud of yourself for an excellent start. Throughout the entire exercise you want to squeeze your core. You'll increase your balance, strengthen your core, and drop some unwanted belly fat. Once again I'll reiterate make sure that you drink water.

Another thing to consider is to stretch out your calves, and ankles. I'll leave some photos of some stretches you can do below.

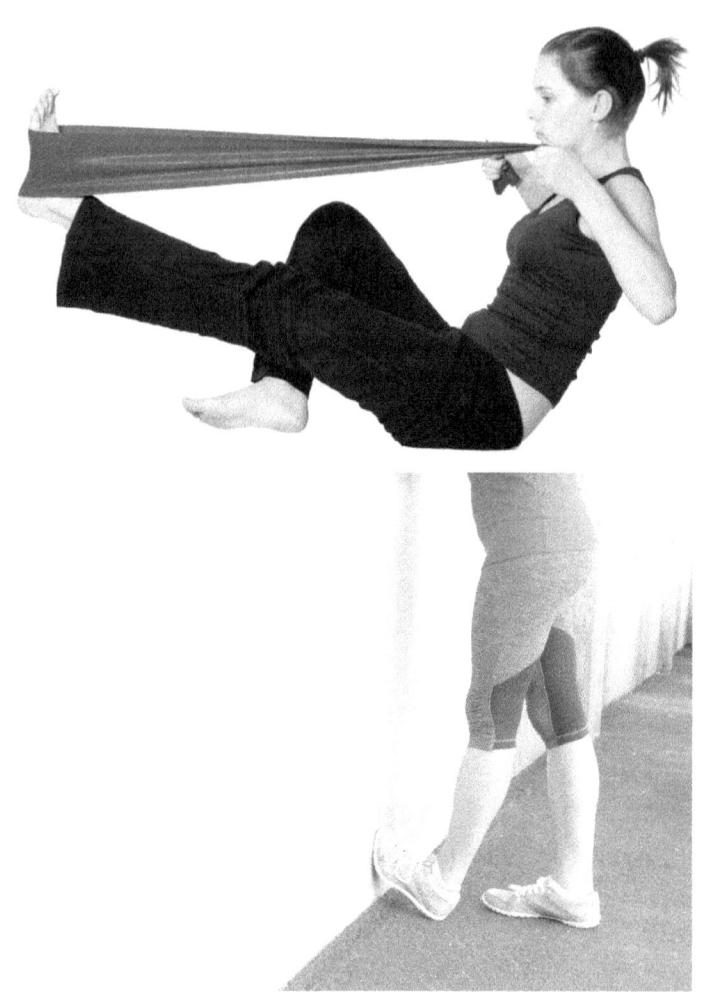

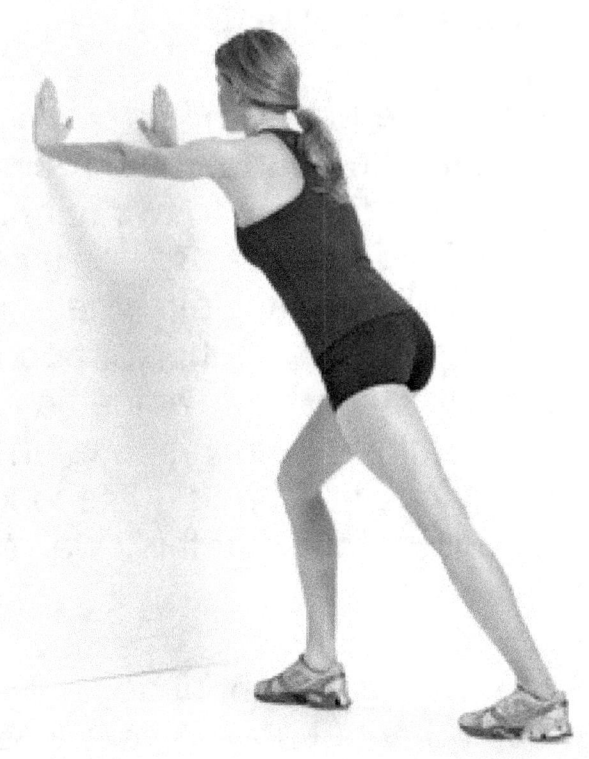

These muscles are slightly temperamental because they're not often worked. That's why you need to stretch, and work them. Your ankles hold up your entire body so you want them to be as strong as iron. For the life of me I can't think of an exercise that works the ankles better than jump roping.

Intermediate

The intermediate program has two steps. Step one start doing an hour of jump roping. Step 2; get your jump time up to two minutes per set. The first thing I did was up my time to 45 minutes. I also upped my jump time to a minute, and 30 seconds. I did this for about 10 to 15 days. Eventually my body adjusted to it, and it was easy for me. I up my time to an hour while still doing one minute, and 30 seconds each set. After about 5 days of this I was able to do 2 minutes each set.

This is the way I went about doing it you can pretty much go about upping your time anyway you want. Grow at your own pace. These are just guidelines you don't have to follow them exactly. The point is to improve. I just want to be very specific about how I went about improving. I found it was easier to increase the time of the session then it was to increase the time of the set. I also found out increasing the time of the session builds up stamina increasing the time of my set. Instead of doing 30 minutes of jump roping one minute each set I could go up to 45 minutes 1 minute each set. Eventually that would get me strong enough to do 1:30 seconds each set.

When I started doing 30 sets of 2-minute jumps everything changed. I started to notice my results come in a lot faster. I started to notice my face slim down, and my waist start to drop. I felt more focused I felt more involved in the exercise. Usually when I exercise I feel like I'm not in the moment. I don't really know how to explain it but I'm pretty sure everyone else will agree with me. Once I got to this point in the jump rope diet I felt in the moment. I was focused, and prepared for the workout. Once I felt that feeling I started to understand why boxers seemed to enjoy this work out so much. It's truly a shared experience between the body, and the mind. That's just my personal opinion I'll let you be the judge.

My wife was especially focused. Usually she's the last one up in the morning but when we reach this point in our training she just had this energy about her. Up and ready before I could even turn the alarm off. That's when I knew we were onto something. After two months the physical results weren't staggering, but we felt sensational. I've never seen my wife have so much energy. Once you reach this point you're ready for advanced level training.

Advance

Things are about to get interesting. When you hit an advanced level it means that you're capable of doing an hour of jump roping three minutes per set. You'll be doing twenty sets 3 minutes each. Now some people go higher honestly I've never done more than a five-minute set. I wouldn't recommend anything more. Even though a man once jumped rope for 36 hours straight with no major issues I'd still be cautious. No one on the planet is as good as Mark Rothstein when it comes to jumping rope.

Now your body is strong, and it requires more resistance. This is where leg weights come in. Now I always say be very careful with leg weights when you're doing cardio exercises. You don't want leg weights that are incredibly loose because it will cause problems. My recommendation would be no more than 5 pounds on each leg. If you can find some leg weights that are well insulated, and don't move around when you jump you can put more weight on. Unfortunately I personally haven't come across any leg weights that fit that description. Leg weights will send you all the way back to the beginning.

Most likely you'll have to do 30 seconds to one-minute sets. Continue to do, and our overall, but be aware that you're set time we'll go down at first. If you can't do an hour do 30 minutes. My set time went down to about a minute when I put 5 pounds on each leg. It was the same with my wife she put 2.5 pounds on each leg. That's what I would recommend for women depending on how strong your legs are. The leg weights make you feel like a beginner all over again, and I love that feeling. It means that the results are going to be amazing, and they were. Adding the leg weights to the workout severely improved my results. Little by little I was able to work back up to 3-minute sets with 10 pounds on my legs.

At this point my wife made a really smart purchase, and bought us some wrist weights. She got 2.5 pounds for each hand. Now we were jumping with 15 extra pounds on us. This brought me down to 2 minutes per set. It didn't take me long to build back up to 3 minutes sets.

If that isn't enough for you than I have a killer of an idea. Why don't you put on a weight vest? This is exactly what my wife said to me right before we bought a 20-pound weight vest. That weight vest changed my life. Once I started jumping with the weight vests on those pounds just dropped off. At first I would only wear the weight vests, and the wrist weights for a total of 25 pounds. This of course took me back to one-minute jumps all over again. With resilience I was able to work back up to 3-minute jumps, and I never felt better.

I remember looking in the mirror, and seeing a totally different guy. It was like I finally broke the mold. I felt like I was stuck for so long so when I got to this point I couldn't do anything, but be proud of myself. No matter how hard the universe tried a negative thought couldn't ruin the moment. I had taken back control. After that feeling I just wanted to up the weight one last time, and add ankle weights in for a total of 35 pounds. Once again I had to go back to one-minute jumps, but I work my way up again.

Another way to increase the resistance is to jump on sand. Not only does it reduce the impact significantly it also makes it more difficult for you to jump. The added resistance makes for a much better workout, and a much safer one. If you add all the extra weight, and jump in the sand you're on a whole new level. Be careful with the weight make sure you don't add more than you can handle. This exercise increases your results significantly, but it's also risky if you're not strong enough. Give your body rest, and make sure you stretch, and keep good form.

Adding the weight helps you build muscle, and burn way more calories. It really made the difference in my training. It's the reason why I was able to lose so much weight. It took a simple exercise, and turned it into weighted cardio.

Motivation

No plan succeeds without motivation. Motivation is the foundation of every major come up or comeback. For some people motivation is like an hourglass eventually all the sand will fall to the bottom. At that point all your motivation will be gone. If that's the case you need to make sure that there's enough sand in that hourglass to carry you to the end.

You need to start off with extreme a amount of motivation. Overtime different things will end up motivating you to push forward. Not only physical results, but also mental results as well. The way that you feel will change which will also motivate you. It might be some time before these results show themselves so you need to have at least 3 months of motivation built up in you before you start this journey. 3 months is long enough to see some results that will than motivate you further. Some people start off a weight loss regimen with only a week's worth of motivation. That's not nearly enough to see any major results. I've heard individuals tell me that I worked out for 2 weeks straight, and didn't see any results. Of course you didn't see any results two weeks isn't nearly enough time for a person to see physical change. That's why I encourage you now to build up as much motivation as you possibly can. You need to understand that some days you're going to wake up, and not want to do this. Some days you're going to wake up, and feel drained, and tired.

Different life circumstances, and events could happen in the middle of your journey. Ah death could occur in your family. A difficult task could come up. A difficult work situation could strain you. You might even lose your job. Through all of this you need to remain motivated, and continue putting your health first. All those things are important, but what's most important is you. For once put yourself first. The best way to put yourself first is to put your health first. Putting your health first is putting your life on a pedestal just a little quote from my wife.

A lot could happen in a three-month time span so beware of the distractions. People mention the small distractions, but it's really the big ones that give people the excuse to stop. If something dramatic happens in their life they feel like it's a big enough excuse for them to stop putting themselves first. For me it was a matter of learning how to cope with different problems in my life through Fitness. Every time something negative would happen in my life I would deal with it by working out. I was able to think clearly on the situation, and make better decisions that way. When you work out your brain works better so you're better capable of dealing with your emotions.

I remember right in the mist of the jump rope diet my grandma died. Now usually an event like this would cause me to backtrack. I remembered what my grandma on my mom's side said to me. She wanted me to take care of myself so that I could live a better life than she did. I know that's exactly what my grandma on my dad's side would have wanted as well. If she knew that I had stopped my fitness she would be upset with me so I continued. More challenging events occurred during this time like me losing my job. Still even during my unemployment I continued my fitness.

My fitness is actually the reason I was able to work a new job. My wife, and I were at the gym jump roping on some yoga mats without the rope when a gentleman approaches us. He wanted to know what we were doing he had never seen anyone jump rope without the rope. Eventually he joined us, and we became great friends. It was through him that I was able to get a new job, and a new workout buddy. Working out is good for keeping a positive mindset that's why it's good to continue your fitness when you're in a negative situation. So no matter what's going on in your life get up grab a friend, and jump.

My motivation was especially high. At no point did I believe giving up was an option. Giving up to me was giving up on my life. My physician made it very clear that if I didn't start taking care of myself I was going to become a diabetic. There was no way I wanted to live like that. The choice was continue being lazy, and become a diabetic, and potentially die or take care of myself, and live a long healthy life. It was pretty much a no-brainer for me. I hope the decision is as clear cut, and dry for you as it was for me. If not you need to find other reasons to be motivated.

Sometimes vanity isn't enough. Most individuals want to get in shape so they can look good, but sometimes that isn't enough. I should say most of the time that isn't enough. That's usually the reason why a lot of people end up in the gym. They want to improve their physical appearance so it has nothing to do with their health. Those who usually stay in the gym are those who are concerned about their health. When you're doing it for vain reasons than your motivation quickly relies on your vanity. If you're not a very vain person then your motivation is going to run out quickly. If you are a very vain individual than your motivation might last a lot longer.

Vanity can be a part of your motivation, but it shouldn't be the driving force. Think about your health, and all the love ones you'll leave behind. Think about your children if you have them. Think about your significant other, and how they'll feel when your health starts to take a turn for the worse. These are solid reasons to be motivated. In my opinion the greatest source of motivation is someone who is just as determined as you are. Having friends to do this with is a powerful source of motivation. If you can get everyone together, and create a sense of camaraderie there's nothing you can't accomplish.

The sense of camaraderie that my wife, and I had is one of the main reasons we were able to finish, and continue our training. If I didn't want to do it she would make me do it. If she didn't want to do it I would make her do it. Eventually we didn't even have to motivate each other anymore it was just second nature. We were going to get up, and we were going to work out. Once it gets to that point you can't lose because now it's a part of your permanent routine like coffee in the morning.

All you need to do is find out how many calories your body needs to maintain its current weight. Eat 500 less calories than that every day. Couple that with the jump rope diet, and you'll be fine.

Vitamin Intake

Let me start this off by saying that by no means am I telling you to buy any of these vitamins. I'm just telling you the vitamins that I used during *The Jump Rope Diet*. I have no idea if they had an effect on my results, but I feel like they're worth mentioning. My vitamin intake during *The Jump Rope Diet* was well rounded. I tried to make sure I covered every single function of my body. Let's start things off with the first vitamin I took.

Ubiquinol is said to be very good for your cardiovascular health, and the last thing I wanted going out on me was my heart because I had high blood pressure. Ubiquinol was a supplement I took to make sure I had a little extra energy. Its supposed to be an incredibly powerful antioxidant it's also supposed to promote energy production as well, and I needed all the energy that I could get. They say it's good for brain health, and protecting the cells from free radicals. To be honest I still use ubiquinol it's much better than Co q-10 because it's easily absorb into the body.

The second thing I kind of supplemented with was *Apple Cider Vinegar With Mother*. I mixed my apple cider vinegar with a teaspoon of lemon juice, eight ounces of water, and made sure to take this every single day at least 2 times a day. I have no idea what kind of effect it may have had on my progression. I just know that it's still apart of my routine to this day. Apple cider vinegar is supposed to promote weight loss. I have no idea if it contributed to my weight loss, but I feel like it's worth mentioning.

The third supplement that I used was *Black Seed Oil*. Black seed oil is supposed to be the God of all supplements. It's supposed to promote health across the board. They say that it's a huge anti-inflammatory. Since pretty much every health problem is caused by inflammation black seed oil is probably the number one vitamin you can use. They say black seed oil is wonderful for cancer prevention, and treatment. They also say it's crucial to liver health. They say that it prevents diabetes. They also say it's great for weight loss which was one of the main reasons why I started using it. They say that it's great for your hair, nails, and skin. They also say that it's wonderful for fighting off infections, and that it's effective against certain strains of superbugs that most antibiotics are not working on anymore. Black seed oil has been studied over, and over again. It's probably one of the most studied supplements on the market so there's some solid science to back up what it does. Still I have no idea if it had a major effect on my workout or not nor do I have any idea if it helped my weight loss.

Another supplement I used was *Grapeseed, Green Tea, & Pine Bark Complex*. The combination of these creates a super antioxidant. The main reason why I was taking it was for energy. The combination of these three things promotes a natural boost in energy. It's not like a caffeine pill or anything like that it's something that works overtime. This is one of those supplements that I don't like running out of I try to make sure that I keep it in stock as much as I possibly can.

I used *Probiotics* because they support your immune system. They're supposed to introduce positive bacteria back into your stomach. This is supposed to help your digestive system, and promote weight loss. I can say that I got sick a lot less often once I start taking the probiotics. Still I started sprinting around the same time so I can't really say which one was super effective.

L-Carnitine was one of the first supplements that I started using. It aids in transforming fat into energy. This is the most important process in weight loss, and energy production. Also it's supposed to aid in muscle building as well. It's supposed to be one of the main elements of muscle building. A lot of bodybuilders use L-Carnitine, and some even say it helps with your overall brain health. Now I don't know if it did any of these things for me I just know during *The Jump Rope Diet* I took it everyday.

Omega-3 Fish Oil is something that I've been taking since I was a kid. It's supposed to support cardiovascular health, and cognitive function. It supports your immune system, your bone health, and your joint health as well. It's also said to support a healthy mood. I don't know if it does any of these things I just know that my mom has been giving me omega-3 fish oil since I was a kid. It's supposed to be one of the most important vitamins on the planet for preserving your body, and promoting overall health.

Vitamin D3 is a supplement I started taking when I realize that I probably wasn't getting enough of it. Vitamin D comes from sun exposure, and since I don't really go outside too often I knew that I probably was vitamin D3 deficient. Vitamin D3 is supposed to support bone destiny, the immune system, and boost absorption of calcium. It's supposed to support neuromuscular function whatever that means. All I know is Vitamin D3 is very important to the body, and if you're not getting enough sunlight than most likely you're not getting enough vitamin D3. Still I have no idea if it had any effect on my performance whatsoever.

Biotin is something that I also supplemented with. It's supposed to be good for your hair, nails, and skin. It's also supposed to support some other viable functions in the body. I guess biotin is one of the key ingredients that your hair needs to grow.

That's one of the main reasons why I was supplementing with it. I will say when I started to use it I did notice a difference in quality in my hair, nails, and the appearance of my skin. It took about three to four months though. Still I'm not sure if that was *The Jump Rope Diet* or the biotin or a combination of both.

Sea kelp was something else that I used. It's supposed to be a source of iodine. Iodine is important for thyroid function. The thyroid regulates a huge amount of functions in your body including your hormonal balance. Your hormonal balance has a huge effect on your energy levels, your mood, and also your weight. If your thyroid isn't functioning properly than most likely you're going to have weight issues. They say this is why the Japanese are so skinny because their diet is rich in iodine. It's because they eat so much seaweed. Still I have no idea if it had any effect on my weight loss.

Garcinia Cambogia is supposed to stop your body from creating new fat. It was featured on Dr. Oz a while ago, and it's supposed to be proven to actually stop your body from creating new fat. Now I'm not sure if it stopped my body from creating new fat all I know is that it was a part of my everyday regimen.

Of course I took a _Multi Vitamin_ because that just makes common sense. Everybody probably takes a multi-vitamin I've been taking one since I was a kid. It's always been apart of my regimen.

African Mango was also something that I included in my supplement regimen. It's supposed to help promote weight loss but there isn't much research behind it to say that it does anything of any kind of significance. Still a lot of people swear by it so I added it to my supplement pile.

I also took _L-Theanine_, and if you're a coffee drinker like me L-Theanine is absolutely essential. It gets rid of that jittery affect that coffee gives you, and makes it a smooth high. It also has some other benefits that might be worth mentioning. Apparently in 1964 Japan approved L-Theanine for unlimited use in all foods. L-Theanine has been linked to relieving stress. It's the key ingredient in green tea, which has been linked to relieving stress.

I'm not endorsing any of these vitamins in anyway. I'm just informing you of the supplements I used during _The Jump Rope Diet._ These supplements may have enhanced my results, and it wouldn't be fair if I didn't mention them. If you choose to take them my best advice is to have a conversation with your doctor. If you want to know the exact supplements that I used than check out my website http://workoutkingrule.blogspot.com/.

Mind Your Diet

If you don't pay attention to what you eat you're not going to be able to accomplish anything. In this situation I'm speaking about eating for energy not eating for weight loss. Remember *The Jump Rope Diet* takes a lot of energy. If you're not eating for energy than you're not going to be able to last for very long. Your body is going to need power so therefore you have to eat the foods that give you the most power. I'm going to give you a detailed example of the type of foods I ate during *The Jump Rope Diet*. You can either mimic this, or find similar foods that might give you the drive you need.

First thing in the morning I made sure to blend a shake. I blended kale, oranges, apples, bananas, blueberries, cranberries, strawberries, and I used apple juice instead of water. I did research on each one of these fruits, and vegetables to make sure that they would give me the optimum performance that I was seeking.

Kale is the healthiest vegetable you can eat. I made sure to put more kale in my shake than anything else. Every single fruit that I mention I used a whole one. I used a whole orange, a whole apple, and ah whole banana. I used about maybe eight cranberries, eight blueberries, and about four strawberries. To be honest after I took the shake in the morning I always would feel wonderful. It was probably the best part of my diet, and a great way to kick off my day. I also had oatmeal because I wanted to make sure that I was getting an extreme amount of fiber.

The combination of these fruits and vegetables gave me an extreme amount of energy. It's probably the one thing that I can attest to my newfound power. It actually boosts my energy level. I don't know if any of my vitamins did anything to actually boost my energy level, but I'm sure my shake did the job. To be honest over time it became even more effective. Most people don't understand that eating healthy is something that takes time to affect your body. Sometimes you'll be able to feel it right away, but a lot of people quit because they don't feel any difference within a few days, or a week. I noticed after a month of taking the shake my overall mood in general changed. Remember I told you I was a very tired, cranky, and moody individual. I was so overweight my body had absolutely no energy whatsoever. When your body has no energy it pretty much ruins everything. You don't want to do anything. I can say that this shake had a profound effect on that mindset, and was a key ingredient in making *The Jump Rope Diet* much more effective. I made sure that I didn't add any sugar to the mix. I also made sure to put cinnamon in my oatmeal. The cinnamon had a profound effect on my health as well. Remember cinnamon is nothing but pure fiber, and fiber is incredibly important to the digestive system. As long as you're going to the bathroom often you're losing weight. You want to make sure you're getting as much fiber as you possibly can. That's why I added apples to the mix because apples are rich in fiber. It's also why I added blueberries to the mix because they're rich in fiber as well. I wanted to make sure that I upped my fiber intake by as much as I possibly could. I also wanted to make sure I was getting a ton of vitamin C.

Vitamin C is the reason why I made sure to add a whole orange. I added bananas to the mix because I wanted to make sure that I was getting a lot of potassium. Bananas are good for Vitamin B6. Vitamin B6 is something that you'll see in almost every natural energy supplement.

Cranberries were just another source of fiber. They have even more fiber than blueberries. They're also packed full of antioxidants. The strawberries were mostly for flavor at first until I started doing more research, and I realize that strawberries were amazing. They can help prevent heart disease, stroke, cancer, high blood pressure, constipation, allergies, asthma diabetes, and depression. Strawberries are ah incredibly effective antioxidant.

Oatmeal is packed full of iron it's probably one of the most iron rich foods out there. It also has an extremely large amount of vitamin B6, magnesium, and vitamin A not to mention 6 grams of protein. Speaking of protein maybe I should discuss what I had for lunch.

Everyday for lunch I would have grilled chicken, beans, and a protein shake. My lunch was all about protein intake. For lunch I wanted to make sure I was getting as much protein in my body as possible. That's why I made sure I had grilled chicken because chicken has an extremely large amount of protein. Chicken is one of the most protein rich meats on the planet, and it's healthier for you than beef or pork. Not to mention it's a lot easier to cook especially if you know how to bake. It's even easier if you have a griller like one of those commercial grillers that drain out all the grease. Everyday when I woke up in the morning I would turn on my rice cooker, and add one cup or two cups of black beans. I chose black beans because they're low in calories. One cup is only 624 calories, and because they are extremely high in dietary fiber, you get 29 grams in one cup. Also because they're high in protein you get 39 grams of protein in one cup. They have an extremely large amount of iron, and ah extremely large amount of magnesium, and calcium so it was an obvious choice. Black beans are ah incredibly healthy super food with 2760 mg of potassium.

The body is supposed to consume at least 30 to 38 grams of fiber every day if you're a man. If you're a woman it's about 25 grams of fiber everyday. So basically one cup of black beans would almost be enough fiber for the day for a man and more than enough for a woman. If you read up on black beans you'll understand just how nutritious they really are. It's one of the most underestimated super foods on the planet. The only substitute that I would ever use for black beans if I didn't have them is quinoa. Quinoa is probably the greatest food on the planet, and the only food that has pretty much all the amino acids that you need. I also made sure that I had a whey protein isolate shake everyday.

For dinner I ate pretty much anything I wanted. I just made sure that I didn't eat any fast food. I completely cut out fast food in general. For dinner I would have a meal with black beans on the side. I would have ground turkey meat, chicken, or fish. I wouldn't have any beef or pork. So I would have some turkey tacos with black beans, and cheese, or I would have some turkey nachos with black beans, and cheese. Sometimes I would eat some salmon, beans, and rice. As long as I added the black beans to the meal I would create any combination I wanted. Eating beans with your meal helps the digestive process. It increases the nutritional value of the meal. I didn't really eat any dessert, but I've never been one to eat dessert anyway so it wasn't a big change for me.

My diet wasn't too extreme it wasn't anything that was impractical. All my food was good it wasn't like I had to eat nasty stuff that I didn't like. When you have to eat a bunch of nasty stuff that you don't like eventually you're going to give up on it. I loved the food I was eating! My shake was delicious, and my oatmeal was always good especially with cinnamon. I never put sugar in my oatmeal I just added cinnamon to it. If I wanted it to taste good I would add some honey. I made sure that I got my honey from the whole food store. Black beans are my favorite especially once you season them with some Lawry's, and some pepper. The grilled chicken was always good because I mean grilled chicken is awesome. Sometimes I would grill chicken and have a chicken black bean salad. It tasted great! My diet gave me energy, power, and change my mood all together. It's the main reason why I was able to go on. If I never changed my diet I would have never saw any positive effects from *The Jump Rope Diet* in the first place because I wouldn't be able to do it. My intention was never to change my diet for weight loss, but to promote energy production. I simply wanted to feel better, and run longer, and this diet accomplished that for me. I didn't find it difficult. If you can find food that has similar nutritious value that you actually find delicious by all means go about it in your own way. I'm just telling you exactly what I did. I don't want to leave any details out because that might be the one detail that contributed to my progression. If you choose to follow my diet to the letter it is more likely that you will see the same results that I did. Maybe you might find some loopholes that I didn't find. You might be able to improve upon the diet. If so please don't hoard information comment, and add your perspective. Tell the people of the dietary changes you implement that worked in combination with *The Jump Rope Diet.* Maybe tells us some of the vitamins that you used in combination with *The Jump Rope Diet*. Share other forms of jump rope training you've tried in combination with *The Jump Rope Diet* that worked for you.

Wrap Up

I have started many fitness programs, and gave up. The only fitness programs that I've ever finished are _The Jump Rope Diet_, _The Kettlebell Cleanse_, and _The Sprint Diet_. That's because these programs work they're clear, and easy to understand. _The Jump Rope Diet_ is clear-cut, and dry. It gave me back my health my energy an my life. I hope that you will find the same success with it. I hope that you will stick to the program regardless of whatever life throws your way. Remember motivation is the number one key to continuing results. You're going to feel amazing you're going to look amazing, and you're going to have a better attitude towards life.

When you take fitness, and health seriously you achieve ah positive mindset. If you feel good you'll think more positively. If you feel bad you'll think negatively. It's all about your default setting. Individuals that are healthy are usually at a positive default setting. Individuals that are not healthy are usually at a negative default setting. Optimism is a great key to life. Children are very optimistic that's why they're always in a great mood. Children believe things are going to get better every single day. That optimism seems to leave us, as we become adults. We are no surer about tomorrow than we are about today.

Adults look at 5 years down the line, and think maybe things will be better. We don't look at tomorrow, and think tomorrow is going to be the greatest day of my life. That's the level of optimism you need to get from point A to point B. You have to believe that what you're doing is working. If you stop believing in the process most likely you won't continue it. The jump rope diet will set you on a great path toward a healthy life. Respect your body, and nurture your mind. Remember what you eat is just as important as how much you exercise. Be cautious of the foods that you put into your body. As long as you lower your calorie intake by 500 you should be just fine.

First you need to understand how many calories your body needs to operate. You can find that information on many websites. Just give them your height, weight, and age than click away. If you are a 200 pound six foot two male you need about 2600 calories to maintain your current weight. To lose weight you would lower your calorie consumption to 2100. Combined with the calories that you lose with the jump rope diet you can expect great results. With that I bid you farewell. Have a happy, and healthy life from the Workout King.

For more fitness gold
Checkout

The Sprint Diet: 3 Min Weight Loss HIIT Training

https://www.amazon.com/dp/B06VTVTZG9

The Kettlebell Cleanse Lose 3600 Calories Ah Day

https://www.amazon.com/dp/B071XTTLXM

My Thanks

Hey I wanted to say

You are awesome for buying my book

If it wasn't for you, then I would be homeless and on the streets

So thank You!

If it wouldn't be a bother, could you leave an honest review about this book at this

Your review will help other readers just like you

www.ingramcontent.com/pod-product-compliance
Lightning Source LLC
Chambersburg PA
CBHW071302280526
45788CB00004B/1820